THE BEHAVIOR OF DOCTORS

Their Health, Their Attitudes, Their Methods

THE BEHAVIOR
OF DOCTORS

Their Health, Their Attitudes, Their Methods

RICHARD W. HUDGENS, M.D.

Professor of Psychiatry
Washington University School of Medicine
St. Louis, Missouri

iUniverse, Inc.
Bloomington

The Behavior of Doctors
Their Health, Their Attitudes, Their Methods

iUniverse books may be ordered through booksellers or by contacting:

iUniverse
1663 Liberty Drive
Bloomington, IN 47403
www.iuniverse.com
1-800-Authors (1-800-288-4677)

ISBN: 978-1-4759-1537-2 (sc)
ISBN: 978-1-4759-1538-9 (ebk)

Library of Congress Control Number: 2012907270

Printed in the United States of America

iUniverse rev. date: 04/25/2012

This book is dedicated to two Missouri family doctors and their husbands—to M. and C., and to L. and S.—with admiration for their devotion to their patients and to each other, and for the knowledge and skill they bring to their work. But especially am I in awe of the courage and endurance that is making them able to prevail through their own trials, and help so many people.

I write with gratitude for the leadership and wisdom of Professors Dr. Charles Zorumski and Dr. Eugene Rubin, who through two books, Demystifying Psychiatry and Psychiatry and Clinical Neuroscience: a Primer, have updated the Washington University message for doctors, students and patients in the 21st century.

Contents

INTRODUCTION

This book is about how physicians behave—at best, at worst, and in-between—with no implication intended that I have behaved better than anyone else. My assumption is that, among other reasons, we went into the field of medicine to help people. We all wrote that on our applications to medical school. Except maybe my college classmate Joel Handelman, who claimed he wrote, "Because M.D. means More Dollars." I didn't believe he put that in his application. He wasn't dumb. This book is about living up to our stated wish to help people. It is about the behavior of doctors in general and psychiatrists in particular, since I am a psychiatrist.

The book is divided into three sections, concerning doctors' health, their attitudes and their methods. Their *health*—good or ill, physical or mental—dominates everything about their behavior, and is here considered first.

Some of their *attitudes* are openly declared in word and action. Some may be unexpressed, their discovery by others depending on observation and intuition. And doctors may be only partially aware of some of their own attitudes, hiding them unreflectively even from themselves. It is a doctor's attitudes—about people, about their work, and about life itself—that say the most about her at any given stage of her always changing life and practice.

The *methods* doctors use in their ever-evolving creation of a framework for living, loving and working, determine finally how effectively they carry out their expressed aim of helping people, assuming they really meant what they said in the first place.

Chapter I

The Health of Doctors—The Good, the Bad and the Ugly

In 1954, when I was in my second year at the Washington University School of Medicine, Evarts Graham, the imposing and revered Professor of Surgery, presented his ground-breaking findings on the connection between tobacco smoking and lung cancer. He and his colleagues had constructed a smoking machine, which extracted the tar from cigarettes. He smeared the tar on the back of mice, who then developed cancer at the site. [This was subsequently memorialized in song in a student show that our class put on: "He painted tobacco juice on the fuzz, said 'Let there be cancer,' and the cancer was."]

So there we were, bright 23-year-old students at a good medical school. Did we all take to heart his convincing lesson ? Some didn't, alas. And none of the big smokers in our class made it out of their 60's.

Move ahead to our 40th class reunion in 1996. Now we were 65, most of us not only still bright, but by this time experienced as well. At the class

1

dinner Carl Lyss, a gastroenterologist never known for reticence, went from table to table and asked each of us and our spouses if we had had our colonoscopies. Five years later, at our 45th reunion, two of our number who had not heeded his advice were absent, being dead of . . . ? Guess what.

All of us, the deceased included, knew that there was just one intra-abdominal cancer, that of the colon, which doctors had a really good chance of catching early, curing, even preventing. Liver? Pancreas? Kidney? Stomach? Good luck. But colon—the great majority of people who die of that one have no real excuse.

It reminds me of the time when 15 years old, I was with my parents on a drive from Houston to San Antonio in the bright dawn of a beautiful spring day. The road crews had not yet made their rounds, and carcasses of armadillos littered the highway. My father commented, "The saddest thing about this is that no other armadillo, viewing this scene, will learn any useful lesson from it. A pity they are so dumb." So let us doctors, above all, not be dumb ourselves. Let's take care of ourselves, or we can't take good enough care of anyone else.

We work within the constraints of our genes, our biologic destinies, which may have programmed us for such things as coronary disease, Alzheimer's, and ovarian cancer. But "life-style choices" can modify that destiny. We can: *not* smoke, *not* abuse substances, *not* eat unwisely. We can get mammograms and colonoscopies on schedule. We can exercise regularly. We all can fly in the face of prevailing genetic winds that impel us in the wrong direction. It's for some of us very hard to do, but so what? What *isn't* hard? We all said we wanted to take care of people, and this is the pathway to doing it more effectively.

Not many are born with the athletic gifts of Chuck Zorumski, now chairman of the department of psychiatry here at the Washington University School of Medicine. He started soccer young and was goal keeper as an undergraduate at St. Louis University the last two years they won the NCAA Division I national championship—in 1972 and '73, Chuck has kept on going, soccer and running, now deep into middle age. He continues to employ his natural gifts, not letting them atrophy in disuse.

More amazing still is my colleague, the psychiatrist Ed Wolfgram, whom God had intended to be a round person, but who defied his stars. *Beginning* in middle age, Ed has engaged in Iron Man competitions well into old age. In these grueling contests of 2.4 miles swimming, 112 miles bicycling and 26.2 miles running—a marathon—he routinely wins against even former Olympians in his age group. He won first place in his age group at age 75 with a stenotic aortic valve and recently came in fourth a few months after it had been repaired in open-heart surgery. He writes books on conditioning, which you can read to your benefit.

These men, with their gifts and their doggedness, are outliers. They are models for us all, though some might say Wolfgram is crazy to put himself through all that.

Dr. Eli Robins was in a class by himself. He was the seventh son of a seventh son, by ancient Jewish legend destined to be gifted as a healer. He was born in Texas in the early 1920's of immigrants from Russia. He rose to become the leader of the group at Washington University that opened the way for clinical psychiatry, long trammeled in the morass of psychoanalytic theory, to become part of the science of medicine. He was the apostle of an evidence-based quest for knowledge in the field, with a question that dumbfounded his challengers whenever they made groundless assertions: "Where are your data?" They had to fall silent, because there were no data to bolster many of their notions. As the late Dr. Theodore Reich, Washington University psychiatrist and geneticist, put it, "The psychoanalytic theorists make up their data as they go on talking."

It is Eli Robins' ill health and his stubborn endurance that are the amazing parts of his story. His greatest achievements and honors came after he had developed multiple sclerosis at age 40, in an era when very little could be done to stem its ravages. He headed the Department of Psychiatry at Washington University from age 41 until ill health forced his retirement when he was 53. He then worked and taught on as best he could till shortly before he died in 1994, when he was 72. His unflinchingly scientific methods of thinking and working, and his kind wisdom, inspired his colleagues and students and his students' students and so on, through several generations in the profession of psychiatry.

Even that was not what I remember most about Eli Robins. He bore his afflictions stoically and accepted in his last years the necessary ministrations of his wife, the late Dr. Lee Robins, and his other care-givers, with an uncomplaining grace. He did not burden his helpers with protestations and apologies for being trouble.

One of the psychiatry professors during my residency at the University of North Carolina told us that he had had three separate psychoanalyses from three different psychiatrists. He began each one while he was in the middle of a depression, and recovered from each episode while he was in that particular analysis. Since the depression recurred after the first two analyses, but had not recurred so far since the third, he concluded that only the third one had been successful and that only the third psychoanalyst was competent. His *post hoc ergo propter hoc* reasoning is still to be found in some psychiatrists. But depressive illness is often marked by spontaneous remissions and recurrences from causes undiscoverable with present knowledge.

That is not the main point of his story. He had gotten help when he needed it instead of waiting till the illness brought destructive consequence to him, his family or his patients. And the help he got—psychotherapy—is as standard first-line treatment for depression today as it was 60 years ago, even with the current availability of antidepressant medications.

Depression usually comes with insight—"Something is the matter with me." Not so mania in many cases—"I'm great! I'm finally my *real self!*" An internist in her mid-40's in the early days of a manic episode, was driving down Lindbergh Boulevard in suburban St. Louis, when she noticed a street sign, which she took as a personal suggestion: "Hey, '*Lindbergh*!' Let's see if this thing can fly!" And off she roared, in and out of traffic, till she blessedly came to a halt when she hit a concrete median. She stepped out into the welcoming arms of two County cops instead of, like Charles Lindbergh, into an adoring throng in Paris.

Such behavior may not be complained about by the people doing it, but by others who are alarmed or threatened by it. So over the course of a bipolar illness it is not easy for a physician who suffers from it to acquire and retain the insight and the discipline to adhere to effective treatment over the years, once he gets such treatment.

In Missouri, as in other states, an Impaired Physicians Program of the state's Board of the Healing Arts identifies, monitors and provides avenues of assistance for physicians who are impaired by mental or physical illnesses. The doctor mentioned above is not typical of those coming to the Board's attention, since cases of drug and alcohol abuse are far more prevalent. The latter are huge problems in society at large, and ultimately depend for their control on insight and sustained adherence to behaviors of recovery by the person himself. But a powerful stimulus to sobriety is provided when the doctor's license to practice depends upon it. Revocation of the license, or threatened revocation, and mandated urine and serum testing by increasingly effective detection methods, can be the wake up call, the "hitting bottom" that some need to get things turned around and assume responsibility for maintaining their own sobriety.

State medical boards also get involved when a doctor's sexual behavior with patients is reported to them. Some cases are out of their helping hands if they have already come before a court as allegedly criminal behavior, like the case of a Missouri psychiatrist sentenced to 133 years in prison for having sexual relations with two of his female patients over a period of several years. The court subsequently found that the women were under the influence of drugs provided by the doctor, which impaired their ability to knowledgeably consent to what was being done to them. Bringing this psychiatrist's behavior to a halt depended on one patient's subsequent complaints, which finally occurred after years of her enduring it.

From time to time a patient has told me a similar story from years past that she says she never told anyone before. Some years ago in an anonymous survey of its membership, the American Psychiatric Association found that 9% of respondents admitted to some degree of inappropriate physical contact with their patients, though not necessarily sexual intercourse. This is unethical by any professional standards. Is it criminal behavior? The late Dr. William Masters, the well-known Washington University sex therapist, said that sexual intercourse between a doctor and his patient, whether or not drugged and whether or not mentally ill, is always rape regardless of the circumstances, because of the disparity of power between the two.

The above convicted Missouri psychiatrist himself said he suffered from "moral insanity" and needed treatment. Is such behavior a mental illness, in and of itself, when other symptoms of psychiatric disorder are not present? And if coercion is not present—if the patient takes the initiative in the matter, for example—is sexual contact between a doctor and a patient, whether a repetitive pattern of behavior or a one-time event, a symptom of illness in the doctor? Sometimes the Board of the Healing Arts says yes, giving the physician the benefit of the doubt and mandating therapy for "sexual addiction," which is not in the American Psychiatric Association's current nomenclature of illnesses. Such treatment is often done in groups and sometimes conducted according to the 12-step model of Alcoholics Anonymous. There are no convincing data, one way or the other, about its effectiveness for sexual misbehavior. Sexual "addiction" is clearly a different animal than addiction to alcohol and drugs. Yet the rigorously followed AA model of daily spiritual exercises and very frequent no-nonsense confrontation by peers in the same fix, can't hurt, and provides a second chance for offenders by a compassionate medical board.

As doctors the state of our own health, good or bad, dominates our attitudes and behavior, helping or hindering us in the work we've chosen to do. We have a substantial degree of control where this precious gift is concerned, despite genetic destiny and the occasional, but inevitable, bad luck.

And finally, whatever way we can manage it, we all should try our best to get "enough" sleep, however many hours that is for each of us. Given the nature of our work, that is at times impossible, and we fall short of our best at such times.

Chapter II

The Attitudes of Doctors

I don't believe that attitudes which spring solely from emotions are trustworthy or helpful in guiding us in the treatment of our patients. If each person's life is exactly as precious as each other person's life—and nothing gives us license to look down from some lofty perch and suppose otherwise—we should not be guided by our emotions, whether of irritation or revulsion or scorn or sexual attraction or whatever. We may not be able to help having these feelings, but we can discipline ourselves not to be ruled by them. The smelly person who won't ever bathe, the young woman with schizophrenia who bashed her baby's head on the sidewalk, the four-pack-a-day smoker who now has lung cancer, the alcoholic woman who repeatedly relapses, the man whose thinks we are the devil, and people whose own decisions, and nothing else, have led them to their current plights: if we have agreed to take care of them, or if they show up in the course of our assigned duties, we take the task on and do what we can. We all said we wanted to be doctors: well, this is what doctors do. We should not "fire" patients for displaying the symptoms of the very illnesses we agreed to treat them for.

11

People with psychiatric disorders will give us many escape routes from the responsibility of caring for them. The best doctors don't avail themselves of such opportunities to let themselves off the hook. Then whom, among those who land in our laps, can we *not* help? People who fire *us* or don't show up for appointments when they are quite competent to decide not to; and people who have something wrong with them that we are not competent to treat them for, and whom we then refer elsewhere. That's it.

Find the Glory and Reflect it Back

What we chiefly bring to each patient, regardless of our specialty or the nature of the affliction, is our *selves*—not medication, surgery, or Band Aids. And how our selves are manifested is through our undivided attention whenever the patients are with us, and our availability for as long as the patients' care is our responsibility. Our attitude is our responsibility, because if we start from the premise that every life is as precious as every other life, then there is a glory in each one of us, including those of our patients laid most low. If we don't see this glory, I believe the fault lies with our limited vision. If we do see the glory, then it is our responsibility to show it to our colleagues, and to the patient herself, blinded as she may be by the black clouds of her depression or other affliction, physical or mental.

There is always something that the doctor can give to his patient at each encounter. It may not be a cure, it may not even be improvement, but there is always something. We should never underestimate our ability to help people, however desperately ill they may be, to "take a sad song and make it better." And the best thing we can do, under any circumstance, is to reflect back the glory we see, the positive, even in its smallest component parts. And to tell the patients what we see.

But is there, in fact, a glory in everyone? People who work in prisons, where many sociopaths are sequestered, and people who have been imprisoned themselves, tell us of remorseless evil-doers they have met there. In the course of medical practice, unless we ourselves work there also, we don't often run into such people. They certainly don't go see a psychiatrist on their own. So I don't know for sure if a glory is in them too. But I believe we are on the most solid ground, and do the most good, if we assume it is there. As long as we don't give them our credit cards or turn our backs, what have we got to lose?

What do we see when we meet a new patient? We focus by necessity on the symptoms and other problems we are called upon to help with. But there is more than that to everyone we meet. There is nothing about a patient's life story and illnesses, past and present, that is not relevant, though degrees of relevance vary. In these life-stories lie the clues to his strengths, his potential, his system of support from his family and others. From all this, if only we take the time to explore it, we can form a view of what is realistically possible, not only with regard to symptom relief, but to overall quality of life as well. The patient's illness and his life experiences may block any possibility of his having such a vision of good health and good times for himself. It's up to us doctors, not ourselves blinded by pessimism, to be messengers of hope.

No hope was seen by one of my professors during my medicine residency, for the 650 pound man admitted to my ward for heart failure. This man in his late 30's spent his days in a gigantic wheel chair selling socks in good weather on a street in Lynchburg, Virginia. The spectacle reminded passers-by of a grotesque parody of Lincoln in his Washington D.C. Memorial. The professor, who had known him for some time before his hospital admission, dismissed him scornfully, "He's a psychopath. He lies about what he eats. He won't diet."

When he died after a couple of days, on a hot Saturday in June, 1958, his body was too big to fit into a refrigerated compartment in the hospital morgue. The pathology staff did not do autopsies on weekends, so when Monday morning came, the odor of his rapidly rotting body filled the air of the Charlottesville, Virginia, city block outside the hospital, compounding his indignity in life with indignity in death.

As it turned out, he had a large tumor of the anterior pituitary which may or may not have accounted for his "psychopathic" eating behavior, but this had never been investigated. The belittling attitude and limited vision of the doctor in charge of his case for some years had blocked such an investigation. He did not see, or if he did, he disregarded, the heroism and endurance of a man cursed with unimaginable bulk and immobility, who soldiered on as best he could against impossible odds, uncomplaining despite it all.

There was a better fate for a 31 year old man with schizophrenia since his mid-teens, homeless on the streets of St. Louis. When he was first brought to a hospital by the police after being found confused and wandering the night streets, the psychiatry service admitted him, gave him medication for a few days then let him go with an appointment for outpatient care, without saying a word to his family.

The next year, at a second hospital, the staff took on the task of dealing with all his problems, not just his auditory hallucinations and paranoia. He was homeless, without health insurance, and for years had been alienated from his family because of his delusions and his threatening behavior. Before he was discharged from this second hospital, he was free of symptoms of his illness and reunited with his family, who had been afraid of him. He now had insurance, a followup appointment to a specific doctor, and a place to stay—with his mother, whom he had tried to sexually assault before his hospital admission, believing she was his girlfriend. Seeing his improvement—the vanishing of his voices and of his paranoia—she had come to understand a lot about his illness after discussions with his doctors, and she became part of the team working for his recovery.

Seven years later he is free of symptoms, taking the antipsychotic medication clozapine (the only one that has been effective), and working in the Independence Center in St. Louis, a comprehensive outpatient recovery program based on the Fountain House model of psychosocial rehabilitation for people with severe mental disorders. Among his jobs there, he guides tours for visitors and prospective patients of the program.

Because of his doctors' broad view of his social and financial needs and his potential, not just a narrow view of only his schizophrenic symptoms, his life has been transformed, and he is helping other people who are in the same state he himself once was in.

WHAT ABOUT "ME"? THE ALIGNMENT OF PRIORITIES.

It's not about us doctors, not ever, insofar as the needs of our patients are concerned. We have our own needs and our own priorities, and we have the responsibility of ordering our lives, protecting our health and conserving our strength. But if we are at work that day, if the patient is right there in front of us, then it's all about him, and we should discipline ourselves not to let our issues intrude upon our duty to him.

Our motive for this exclusive focus on the patient's needs when we are with him—in person, on phone, or on-line—should be the result of an intellectual decision that it's our job, not dependent upon some soaring emotion of affection or pity we feel at the moment. Sometimes the only emotion we feel will be annoyance, when we are called at 3 a.m. after a tiring day. We can't trust our emotions to guide us. Nor should our behavior be guided by an assessment that this patient is worse off than we are—impoverished, homeless, bereft, whatever. Sometimes that will not be the case. We all eventually will have great sorrows, if we haven't already: miscarriages, cancer, the loss of the dearest person in our life, or other tragedies. Even then, if in the midst of our troubles we are nevertheless at work, or on call for our patients, then it's about them only, not about us at all.

WHO DO WE THINK WE ARE?

We doctors work this out as we grow in our lives and our profession. Over the millennia it has often been said that people do the most good and find the most enduring peace if they see themselves as servants—in a doctor's case, servants of her patients, of her family, and of science. This accords with the tenets of every major religion on earth, regardless of doctrinal differences and animosities among religious organizations. Reverence for life, care for the widow and orphan, rejection of greed and envy as bases for behavior, are at the heart of Judaism, Christianity, Islam, Hinduism, Buddhism, despite whatever extra baggage the devotees of those traditions may have loaded onto their fundamental principles over the years.

I believe that as a physician faces each patient in his care, in full knowledge of his own imperfections as a doctor, he should assume that he may be the best doctor this patient will ever see. He should pass the responsibility on to another doctor, or share it with another, when a solution to the problem is clearly beyond his knowledge and capabilities. But otherwise he should ask himself, as the case proceeds, "If I don't care, who will? If I don't try, who will? If I give up, who won't?"

Viewing all the sadness and injustice that the world contains, we may be tempted to discouragement that we can fix so very little of it, or even fix such a small proportion of the mess in one patient's life. No matter how expert we are, nor how widely our authority extends, our power to fix things is still weak in the face of all that needs doing. Of course it is, as in every human enterprise. We do the best we can, holding ourselves to a high but achievable standard, concentrating on the process of helping in the immediate present, unfazed by the size of the task.

THE BOUNDARIES OF OUR JOB: HOW FAR DO WE GO?

Our caring for the patient and his welfare can be limitless, but our actions on his behalf, however well meaning, must have limits. Here I have learned hard lessons.

I'm very activist. I try to make it happen, be the patient's advocate, call his boss with his permission, round up his family with his permission, make a home visit when it is in the patient's best interest and the only reasonable alternative. When I was a psychiatrist in the Air Force, a year out of residency training, I went to the home of a paranoid patient with whom I had a good relationship, and coaxed out of his hand the shotgun with which he intended to shoot his wife, when the alternative was to call the police—which he said, and I believed, would have precipitated a tragedy.

19

I think that was a good move. But sometimes I have overstepped my proper boundaries.

When I was a resident in medicine, a woman 90 years old and very obese was admitted to my ward with what turned out to be e-coli meningitis. I was up all night with her, did a lumbar puncture, got a nurse to special her, gave fluids and antibiotics, never left her side. She died in the morning, and when her daughter soon arrived to get the news from me, the nurse who had specialed her intercepted the daughter before I could break the news, to present the bill for her services. I was furious. I took the nurse by the arm and hustled her to the nursing service office to complain about this. Well, guess who got in trouble—for touching the nurse and hauling her to what I thought was judgment. The Professor of Medicine, William Parsons, straightened me out about my inexcusable crossing of personal boundaries, and pointed out my duty to lead as a voice of reason, not an angel of vengeance. I had made it my fight. It was not. It could have cost me my job.

We do the most good if we don't assume there are villains. The "schizophrenogenic mother," once widely blamed in some parts of the psychoanalytic community for allegedly raising her children in such a way that they later developed schizophrenia, has not yet been found. Perhaps she is in hiding with Bigfoot.

Of course there *are* villains—abusive spouses, cruel mothers, and so forth. But in my experience, in most cases such people are not lurking behind cases of depression, bipolar disorder, schizophrenia and so forth. Some psychiatrists just *must* find a villain. Like the psychiatrist in Chicago whose "aha moment" came when a depressed freshman girl at Northwestern University, who had been perfectly well till two months before, told him that she and her twin brother had engaged for awhile in mutual sex play when they were 10 or 11 years old. In that inexperienced psychiatrist's view, this rather routine history was promoted to a par with coerced sex, or even rape, between a parent and child, and assumed to account for any psychological troubles that subsequently ensued in the young woman's life.

I still have to remind myself not to too readily identify people as villains. A couple of years ago, I was the subject of a complaint to the Missouri Board of Healing Arts, after I had chewed out, by phone and most intemperately, the husband of a patient who had been cruelly treated by him. On another occasion, my department head Chuck Zorumski came down on me for launching a minor campaign to get canned a verbally abusive counselor in the Chemical Dependency Program, who was not in my chain of command. Wait till he hangs himself, said wise Zorumski, don't make yourself the issue. And shortly after that, he did get himself fired, with no help from me.

A doctor's strong point, caring intensely and going the extra mile, can be his undoing if he makes the fight his own crusade without proper regard for boundaries and for the person he is trying to help. Without such a regard, the doctor can become more trouble than help, and set a bad example, besides, for the people he is supposed to be teaching, which in my own case, would be inexcusable for a professor in a medical school.

The days of the arrogant doctor who gets away with it seem to be passing. Hospital boards and patients, less docile and more informed than in times long past, are less and less likely to put up with it. A few dinosaurs linger on; but the meteor has landed, and I hope their days are numbered.

I believe that women have a lot to do with things going in the right direction, though Utopia will never be reached. There were only three—among 95 men—in my graduating class from medical school. Now among the Washington University medical students it's a ratio of about 50-50. Men behave better when there are women who are peers and bosses, not just subordinates, in the work place. And the women set an example by being in general more compassionate and better listeners than are men. Published data support this.

CHAPTER III

DOCTORS' METHODS OF WORKING

There was a brief time in the early days of America's involvement in World War II, as chronicled by William Menninger, when more troops were being evacuated from war zones and discharged for psychiatric symptoms than were currently being brought into the military through the draft. It was also feared, based on World War I history, that chronic disability of the discharged soldier might then ensue. Whether that was true or not, it was clearly a practice which, for reasons of military necessity, could not be continued.

This was most notable in the North African campaign of 1942-3, when green American ground troops first encountered the hardened veterans of Erwin Rommel's Afrika Korps. The incident wherein General George Patton berated and slapped a soldier who had been hospitalized for "shell shock," was dramatized in the movie about him.

There began the practice of ordering a brief respite from combat while the soldier remained in the forward area, sometimes with the temporary addition of sedatives, followed by a return to full duty. This worked well enough to become standard practice. And this method also made the movies, in a 1963 film with the late Gregory Peck, "Captain Newman, M.D."

No such niceties were observed in the Red Army of the Soviet Union in World War II, whence no one was ever discharged from duty for psychiatric illness. During the battle of Stalingrad the advancing Russian troops had at their backs sharp-shooters of the state security service, who killed those who turned around and retreated, the best deterrent of all. As amplified in the war novel "Catch-22," it's not crazy, but normal, to fear combat. People go ahead and enter combat through loyalty to the comrades in their units, attention to the task at hand, and fear of the consequences of disobedience.

It must have been so from time immemorial. In World War I my father was a captain in the U.S. Infantry. In one action he was readying his company to go "over the top"—out of their trench to advance on the waiting Germans, to walk behind a covering barrage from American howitzers. The barrage was timed to lift just as the infantry reached the German trenches. One of his men lay curled up and quivering with fear, refusing to go. My father told me that he drew his pistol, thrust it in the soldier's abdomen and said, "Get over the top, you yellow-bellied son-of-a-bitch or I'll kill you right here." The man was less afraid of the Germans, who would probably not have killed him, considering the odds, than of my father, who told me later that he certainly *would* have killed him. The soldier's decision made good sense. Both went over the top, and both survived the action. It was behavior therapy for a phobia, 1918 Western Front version.

THE TYRANNY OF TIME CONSTRAINTS AND THE INCOMPLETENESS OF OUR KNOWLEDGE

We don't know enough, and too often we don't have time enough, to adequately make use of what we do know, in order to best help our patients. What can be done about this?

Not all doctors, but the most effective ones, learn how to organize the work confronting them each day, ordering the priorities. They try to get what they have learned is enough sleep for them, either with consecutive hours or with interval naps during their working hours. They discipline themselves to not waste motion during work and to not let pile up the paperwork like charting duties and forms to be filled out: procrastination—threatening to make them like hoarders, those little old ladies eventually found buried in their homes along with multiple dead cats, under a mountain of rubbish.

It helps if we regard everything we do on behalf of patients—talking with them and their families, writing prescriptions, filling out those endless forms, and so forth—as having equivalent value in the process of helping them. All tasks, however tedious, have that same goal. Some of our work is enjoyable, some tedious and no fun at all. So what? Whining does not become us.

And knowledge, about patients' illnesses and their treatment, and about non-medical matters relevant to an individual patient, is so instantly at hand that there is no justification for our not availing ourselves of it. There is no excuse, in 2012 as I write this, for a busy practitioner of medicine not to have a phone with access to a huge treasure trove of information and communication links to people who can help her out. She can even get her phone to send her updates relevant to her individual practice. As her career moves forward, a physician can get better and better at what she does, if granted the blessings of good health and a long life. And even with significant health issues she may be able to so order her life and work that she does others a world of good.

Two women come to mind—one 41, whom I have treated for five years, and the other 57, whom I have treated since she was 25. They are practitioners of family medicine, that most demanding of specialties, in different Missouri towns. They have struggled since their teens with vicious depressive illnesses which at times have nearly killed them. Yet, here they still are, working every day with knowledge, skill, compassion and dedication beyond those of most of their peers. Each has a husband, equally bright and dedicated, who has stuck with her through their most dark, turbulent and frightening episodes of depression, remaining loyal, never going away, never deviating from the path of loving care.

Imagine what role models of courage and love these couples are to their children. Imagine what an inspiration they are to me, and what they have taught me. What a blessing it is to have a job where I run into people like this.

We should always give something to our patients beyond carrying out a narrowly-defined duty to treat their illnesses. One of the things we can give is our gratitude for what they have taught us, and for the trust they have shown in opening their lives to us, as I do now in dedicating this book to the above two couples and their children. And their little dogs too.

BEGINNING THE PROCESS OF HELPING A NEW PATIENT

Every new patient is an undiscovered country, no matter how much like us he may be, and no matter how much we know about him before we meet him. We should assume nothing and make use of every available source of information—written records, families and so forth.

Our attentive, caring presence has healing power, even in the most afflicted patients. And not for the patients only, but for their distressed families as well.

It is a serious mistake, and bad for our patients, if we regard them or their family members as potential adversaries in a law suit. If we do, they may read it in our words and manner and in the tone of our voice, widening any trust gap between us and them and increasing the odds, however small, that they will be unforgiving of our inevitable mistakes and the occasional, but also inevitable, bad outcomes.

Doctors' Behavior: "The Old Days" and 2012

Reflecting back over the 60 years since I first came to the Washington University School of Medicine, I hardly ever have a pang of nostalgia. Things are far from perfection here, but on the whole, they are also far better than they were in 1952.

When a real time machine is built, I'll book a trip to the India of 500 B.C. to meet the Buddha, and to Israel 2000 years ago to see and listen to Jesus in the flesh. I'll also go to Washington D.C. in 1804 and enter the lottery for a chance to have dinner in the White House with Thomas Jefferson (after making a contribution to his re-election campaign), hoping for a better result than my failed bid to be selected this current election year for dinner with the Obamas. But I would not go back to the St. Louis of 1952, the Charlottesville VA of 1956, or the Chapel Hill NC of 1959.

Back then I had to hurry hundreds of yards, in person, to find a journal article or an x-ray or lab report. Back then it was often difficult or impossible to contact someone whose help was needed, right away, for a critically ill patient. Back then the inpatient divisions at Barnes Hospital were racially segregated. Black male patients, medical and surgical, were placed in division 0400, the initial zero denoting that the unit was underground. It had no windows and no air-conditioning, just big fans. Black women patients were in division 2300 on the second floor, but in a unit surrounded by other units, just as windowless and steamy as 0400.

There were two city hospitals in St. Louis—one for white people, one for black people. If you were found down on a street, the ambulance took you not to the nearest hospital, but to the one for people of your "race", which was determined by the color of your skin. Until 1957, that is, when a man of indeterminate color was found unconscious near the black city hospital. He looked white to the ambulance driver, who took him to the white hospital. In that emergency room, someone decided he was really black and sent him back to the black hospital. He died on the way. The cruel stupidity of the policy was finally revealed publicly, and changed.

No, I would not get off the time machine to revisit the 1950's.

The era did have some eccentric and colorful characters, their likes seldom seen today, who were good doctors nevertheless. Oscar Swineford, an internist at the University of Virginia, rode two hobby horses—the search for foci of infection at the roots of teeth and in the sinuses, and the search for high titers of brucella antibody in the serum. Brucellosis was contracted from eating unpasteurized milk, rarely available even in those days. We on the hospital's house staff ordered many teeth and sinuses x-rayed and drew much blood and prescribed many antibiotics. The disorders whose cause Swineford was seeking and treating were arthritis and many other disorders now thought to have an autoimmune basis. We thought Swineford a bit of a nut on the subject, and recounted often his behavior when he had been a pilot during World War I and flown his fighter plane under a bridge on the Rivanna River near Charlottesvillle. Today it is clear that his quest was ahead of its time, and that he was getting onto some things which immunologists would later pursue with success for their patients.

Despite what we then regarded as his eccentricities, we younger doctors respected Swineford for, and profited by, his example of meticulous histories and physical examinations. He was a role model to me in another very important respect: he took on the toughest cases, sent to him by doctors far and wide who had given up on them, and he himself never gave up. He worked us hard, and we griped. But we learned a lot from him about what it meant to be a doctor, and I remember him with gratitude.

Not so another figure from the past. This neurologist at Washington University, who died in his early nineties 20 years ago, was widely praised as a "sharp clinician" and endowed a professorship at the medical school. But during my years as a medical student and as a young member of the faculty, his behavior set a dreadful example, which for me canceled out his virtues.

For he was cruel, sexist and outspokenly racist. In his case descriptions to us he spoke of patients with crudeness and disrespect. Once on rounds with my colleague George Murphy, and in the very presence of the patient, a physician with Huntington's disease, he described the inevitable hopeless progress of this terrible affliction, an ordeal of deterioration seeming endless to the sufferer, through physical helplessness to dementia to death.

He spoke as if the patient wasn't even there; and the next day he truly *wasn't* there, having killed himself after the presentation of his case.

This neurologist patted female nurses on the buttocks—and got away with in back in those days. His racism was unabashed. When I was a student walking with him down a hospital corridor one day, we came to a door to the outside, which he opened with his foot, explaining to me, "I have misophobia, fear of germs. I never touch the handle of this door—niggers use it all the time."

The wife of another faculty member, Herb Rosenbaum, happened to get on a hospital elevator with this neurologist. A black woman with a mop and a pail was cleaning the elevator. He remarked quite aloud, "Do you notice how many niggers there are, everywhere we go around here? It's impossible to get away from them." Young Mrs. Rosenbaum wanted to disappear through the floor.

He was inflicted on psychiatric patients as well, since he was a neuro-psychiatrist. When one of his hospital patients was making no progress, he would enter as his only note in the chart that day a Biblical citation: "Hebrews 13:8". If you looked it up you would find, "Jesus Christ, the same yesterday, today and forever." The name, Jesus

Christ, being here used as an expletive, not an invocation. So to this neurologist's other character traits and examples for the edification of students and residents, add public irreverence. His clinical notes are still to be found today imbedded in the microfilmed records of Barnes-Jewish Hospital.

None of this behavior would be tolerated today at Washington University or any other medical school, the wealth of the perpetrator notwithstanding.

OVERSIGHT OF DOCTORS: THE 21ST CENTURY REALITY

In the same way that the authors of the United States Constitution learned that public officials needed a system of checks and balances to guard against an untrammeled slide into tyrannical behavior, so have people concerned with the practice of medicine learned that doctors, both as individuals and as organized groups, cannot altogether be trusted to govern themselves. Increasingly, courts, state legislatures, state medical boards, the American Medical Association, specialty boards, the Federal government, hospitals and the national bodies governing them, insurance companies and so on, have moved to oversee doctors' behavior, to protect patients from dangerous and wasteful practices, and from malpractices due to doctors' ignorance, apathy, greed or misbehaviors of any sort that may occasionally arise.

The result of this is that the days of the cowboy have ended, and though many doctors, the oldest ones in particular, complain about the resulting paperwork and re-certification demands, the old days are not coming back. Too bad? Well, guess what, it's not about us doctors at all, it's about our patients.

Professor Michael Jarvis, Vice Chairman for Clinical Affairs and Director of Inpatient Psychiatry in our department, who is also trained in forensic psychiatry, occupies an important position of leadership for which he is well suited in this modern climate of oversight of doctors and the corralling of the cowboys among us. We owe much to his diligence and wisdom. He has taught me a lot that I needed to know, and he keeps on teaching us all. In his unique way, he has even improved my penmanship.

Conclusion

This book about doctors' health, attitudes, and methods of working is written for physicians and for those on their way to becoming physicians. The illustrative anecdotes are true stories, but I have omitted the names of doctors whom I have criticized. I hope the book will be helpful in the care of patients.

Richard W. Hudgens, M.D.

Professor of Psychiatry

Washington University School of Medicine

www.ingramcontent.com/pod-product-compliance
Lightning Source LLC
Chambersburg PA
CBHW050349290526
45785CB00006B/2698